Using the Internet for Health Information

Legal Issues

Stephen J. Schanz, JD, LLM

Using the Internet for Health Information
Legal Issues

© 1999 by the American Medical Association
Printed in the USA.
All rights reserved.

Internet address: http://www.ama-assn.org

Cover photo © Tom Ellicott Photography. Used with permission. All rights reserved.

No part of this publication may be reproduced, stored in a retrieval system, or transmitted, in any form or by any means, electronic, photocopying, recording, or otherwise, without the prior written permission of the publisher.

This publication is distributed with the understanding that neither the publisher nor the author is engaged in rendering legal, financial, medical, or other professional advice. The author has exerted his best efforts to ensure the accuracy of the contents of this book. However, the material set forth herein is for informational purposes only. Original source materials should be consulted prior to reliance on cited sources to ensure that relevant material has not been repealed, modified, or changed since the date of original compilation. Finally, if legal, medical, financial, or other professional advice is required, the services of a competent professional should be sought.

Additional copies of this book may be ordered from the American Medical Association. For order information call toll-free 800 621-8335. Mention product number OP317399.

ISBN 0-89970-977-X

BP38:98-1484:1.5M:6/99

About the Author

Stephen J. Schanz, JD, LLM, is president of Legamed, Inc, a medical-legal information company in Raleigh, North Carolina. He received a JD from Pepperdine University School of Law in Malibu, California, and an LLM in Health Law from Loyola University School of Law in Chicago, Illinois. Licensed to practice law in Michigan and North Carolina, Mr Schanz is also an Adjunct Associate Professor at East Carolina University School of Medicine and Professor of Business & Economics at Meredith College, where he is the Director of the Masters of Health Administration Program.

Acknowledgments

The author wishes to thank Barry B. Cepelewicz, MD, JD, for his valuable assistance in reviewing this manuscript. Mr Cepelewicz is an attorney in the health care group of Meiselman, Farber, Packman & Eberz, PC, in Mt Kisco, New York.

The author also wishes to thank the Mayo Clinic and America's Doctor, Inc, for graciously permitting the inclusion of their Web site disclaimers in the Appendix of this book. Additionally, the author is indebted to Marsha Mildred, Jean Roberts, Denise Bryson, Rosalyn Carlton, and Patrick Dati, all with the American Medical Association, for their valuable assistance in the development, editing, production, and marketing of this publication.

Table of Contents

Prologue   vii

Section 1   General Legal Issues in the Electronic Information Age   1
- The Growth of the Internet   1
- Cyberjurisdiction   2
- The Patient-Physician Relationship   6
- Medical Records   7

Section 2   Health Information on the World Wide Web   11
- Accuracy and Timeliness of Information   11
- Authentication and Verification   12
- Interactive Web Sites   13
- State Medical Licensure   18

Section 3   Issues in Health Care Communication via E-mail   21
- Using E-mail to Communicate Health Care Information   21
- Confidentiality and Privacy of E-mail   21
- E-mail Between Patients and Providers   23
- Incorporating E-mail Technology   26
- Mailing Lists and Newsgroups   26

v

Section 4	Strategies for Cyberspace Risk Management	31
	Encryption 31	
	Malpractice Insurance 32	
	Rationales for Disclaimers 35	
	The Use of Disclaimers in Health Care Web Sites 36	
	The E-mail Agreement 40	
Conclusion		43
Appendix A	Warning to Internet Users From Minnesota Attorney General	45
Appendix B	HCFA Internet Security Policy	53
Appendix C	Disclaimer Used on America's Doctor Web Site	65
Appendix D	Disclaimer Used by Mayo Clinic	75

Prologue

This book will discuss the myriad legal issues involved in the transmission and dissemination of electronic medical information via the Internet. Concepts relating to international transmissions, however, will be excluded from discussion, as well as such intellectual property matters as copyrights and trademarks. Both are too extensive to cover in this publication.

The scope of legal issues stemming from the electronic communication of health information is enormous. For purposes of this publication, Internet health communication will be divided into 2 distinct categories: the use by health care providers of Web sites through which the public can search and/or download information and the use of e-mail for health care matters. Though the 2 categories do have similarities, their distinctions warrant separate analyses.

The continuing development of the Internet, in terms of both Web sites and e-mail, offers enormous potential for health care providers, patients, and consumers desiring health-related information. Expanded use, however, potentially triggers legal issues of which a responsible health care provider or patient should be cognizant. Although the discussion of potential legal issues affecting providers, consumers, and patients may, at times, be worrisome, it is important to view these concerns within their proper context.

The use of the Internet and e-mail for the exchange of health information generally, and patient-specific information in particular, offers significant advantages for the quick, inexpensive, and convenient transmission of health care information:

- Information can be retrieved, or messages sent and read, at times convenient for the retriever.
- The sender does not have to be available simultaneously with the reader.
- Changes in time zones and individual schedules are no longer a barrier to communication.
- The expenses associated with sending e-mail and downloading information off the World Wide Web are minimal.

Despite such advantages, the use of e-mail and the Internet as means of transferring health information presents legal issues of which providers and consumers alike need to be aware. The responsible use of Internet technology for the transmission of patient-specific data, especially, requires consideration of the legal issues discussed in this book. Recitation and discussion of legal issues should not, however, be construed as a barrier to the implementation of such technology. Rather, the recognition of legal concerns should serve as a catalyst for providers to work hand in hand with legal counsel, insurance carriers, hospitals, employers, and health care institutions in an effort to use modern technology within acceptable legal boundaries. Building an information system that takes into consideration such important legal issues as privacy and confidentiality will yield better results for both providers and consumers.

Section 1
General Legal Issues in the Electronic Information Age

The Growth of the Internet

The growth of the Internet has been, in many ways, both an advantage and a disadvantage. The ease with which information can now be transferred 24 hours a day, 7 days a week, has proved to be valuable to both health care entities and other businesses. Some estimates predict that at least 40 million people are connected to the Internet and that almost 20 new users log on every 30 seconds.[1] Additionally, the US government believes the number of Internet users will increase to 200 million by 1999.[2]

Both governments and private industry have been involved in the rapidly expanding growth in Internet use. The US government has been a leader in the use of Web sites for its various agencies and offices; the Department of Health and Human Services (HHS), the Health Care Financing Administration (HCFA), the Food and Drug Administration (FDA), and the White House all have Web sites available to the public. In fact, HHS operates more than 60 central Web sites on 8 separate domains.[3] It has also been estimated that there are more than 10,000 health care-related sites on the World Wide Web.[4] Several states, including Wisconsin, Utah, and

---

[1] Pergament D. Internet psychotherapy: current status and future regulation [note]. *Health Matrix.* Summer 1998;8:235;footnote 2.
[2] Id.
[3] Public Health News and Notes. DHHS consumer health on the Web. *Public Health Reports.* 1997;112:451.
[4] Id.

Minnesota, are also active in Internet health information. MedNet, for instance, is state operated:

> The Minnesota Health Data Institute (MHDI), formed as a public/private partnership, operates MedNet, a shared, secured nonproprietary information frame relay network, through which providers, payers, employers, policymakers, consumers, and others can communicate with each other electronically. Participants have used MedNet primarily for its network routing and addressing services, which facilitate the exchange of administrative, clinical, and analytical health information.[5]

Laws relating specifically to the Internet are virtually nonexistent at the present time, however, in comparison with the extensive bodies of law dealing with other areas. Analyses and comparisons of how existing laws may affect use of the Internet for health information are therefore necessary. Because Internet use continues to grow at an incredible rate, it is probably inevitable that legal issues will arise from Internet use for health matters, especially in light of the fact that courts address new issues only after a case or controversy has arisen. In many ways, the development of case law lags behind technological developments such as the Internet. As a result, an awareness of existing legal concepts that may be relevant to issues of Internet use is essential to providers.

Cyberjurisdiction

One of the most profound legal questions confronting the modern use of the Internet involves the identification of "where" the Internet—commonly referred to as cyberspace—actually is. Since the Internet is a network of interconnected computers around the

---

[5] Mendelson DN, Salinsky EM. Health information systems and the role of state government: a taxonomy and evaluation of state government efforts on the health information frontier. *Health Affairs.* May-June 1997.

globe, identifying where electronic information or messages "are" is virtually impossible. For example, if a Washington, DC, health care association maintains a Web site containing clinical information via an Internet service provider (ISP) located in Georgia, where is the information located when viewed by a patient in California? Arguably, the information can be seen as residing in any of the 3 states. For purposes of the law, however, this unresolved issue presents perplexing, and often troublesome, problems.

Most states have designed statutes to protect their citizens from improper or unscrupulous business practices. Additionally, every state governs a host of issues, including taxation, business and trade practices, crimes, confidentiality, etc, using a criminal code that specifies certain acts to be illegal and mandates punishment for violations. Current uncertainty over the location of information in cyberspace (or "where" the Internet is located), however, generates ambiguity regarding the applicability of particular state laws. At a minimum, those using the Internet for such business purposes as the dissemination of health-related information or promotion of health-related products should carefully research whether particular state laws affect their use of the Internet.

Consider, for instance, the recent action of the Minnesota Attorney General. That office posted a "Warning to All Internet Users and Providers" (see Appendix A) outlining the position taken by the Minnesota Attorney General regarding the applicability of its state laws to those communicating with Minnesota residents via the Internet. Minnesota's position is that use of the Internet to attract commercial transactions with its residents can submit the message originator to the jurisdiction of Minnesota law and Minnesota courts. In relevant part, the posted message states:

> THIS MEMORANDUM SETS FORTH THE ENFORCE-
> MENT POSITION OF THE MINNESOTA ATTORNEY
> GENERAL'S OFFICE WITH RESPECT TO CERTAIN
> ILLEGAL ACTIVITIES ON THE INTERNET.
>
> PERSONS OUTSIDE OF MINNESOTA WHO TRANS-
> MIT INFORMATION VIA THE INTERNET KNOW-
> ING THAT INFORMATION WILL BE DISSEMINATED
> IN MINNESOTA ARE SUBJECT TO JURISDICTION
> IN MINNESOTA COURTS FOR VIOLATIONS OF
> STATE CRIMINAL AND CIVIL LAWS.

The posting then recites excerpts of various Minnesota criminal and civil statutes as a way of explaining the rationale behind the Minnesota Attorney General's position. Included with these points are scenarios in which a person can be convicted of a crime:

- an offense is committed, in whole or in part, within the state;
- a person outside the state aids, causes, or abets another to commit a crime within the state; or
- a person outside the state "intentionally causes" a result within the state which is prohibited by state criminal law.

A similar rationale is put forth as establishing jurisdiction in civil cases: namely, causing something to occur within the state which is normally a regulated activity (cited examples include the necessity for an Indian tribe to register political ads in a newspaper pursuant to state ethical laws even though the "action" occurred on the reservation), and participation via the Internet in activity that is prohibited by the state, like gambling. The placing of bets or purchase of lottery tickets through the Internet by a resident of a state that prohibits gambling may subject that person to the jurisdiction of the state that prohibits the activity.

In a theoretical sense, responsible use of the Internet for the transmission or dissemination of health information requires that the user be cognizant of various state laws that may impact the intended activity. Web sites that (1) contain health care information or (2) promote or advertise health care products or services may be subject to the jurisdiction of many state laws addressing taxes, advertising, various consumer protection acts, deceptive trade practice acts, etc. Vigilance is likely to be an evolving process as states continue to formulate policies and laws governing Internet transactions and related use.

Providers of Internet-based health information should also consider some of the uncertainties that may arise in disputes involving Internet use. A Web site offering information that a user subsequently asserts is inaccurate, or a site offering some degree of interactivity like a bulletin board for the posing of questions with resultant answers, may present serious legal questions regarding:

- which state law governs a site,
- where proper jurisdiction to resolve disputes is located,
- whether the clinician providing answers is deemed to be "practicing" medicine and thus would be required to be licensed in the relevant state, and/or
- whether the sponsoring company is considered to be "practicing" medicine in violation of applicable state laws.

These are in addition to such nonmedical issues as mandates against false and misleading advertising, etc.

As is discussed later in this book, the degree of Web site interactivity appears to substantially affect how courts determine state jurisdiction. Passive sites often are not enough to trigger personal jurisdiction, while a highly interactive site tends to heighten the risks.

The Patient-Physician Relationship

Practitioners disseminating information through electronic interaction with consumers need to exercise caution to avoid the unintentional creation of a patient-physician relationship. Limiting the degree of interaction and data input by the user, together with disclaimers, can go a long way in effectively communicating the sponsor's intent. Many sites are designed for informational purposes only and clearly state as much on the first page.

Even with disclaimers, however, site sponsors should be vigilant about the extent to which they interact with users lest they risk a user's claim that the patient-physician relationship has been established. In the event a court finds the patient-physician relationship to exist, the dynamics of the resulting legal responsibilities change considerably. In such cases, issues relating to the professional standard of care, medical record creation and retention, privacy and confidentiality, and the applicability of medical malpractice insurance coverage all become relevant to physician and patient alike.

In a legal sense, patient-physician encounters are often based on oral contracts or conduct the parties reasonably believe will trigger the patient-physician relationship. Unfortunately, there is no universally recognized "bright line" that determines, in all situations, whether the patient-physician relationship has been created. As is typical with the law, each case is fact dependent. The use of the Internet to communicate with health care consumers gives rise to innumerable potential factual scenarios, many of which the law has yet to address.

The patient-physician relationship is central to a determination of the scope of duty owed to a patient. Because technology is always changing, no definitive case outlines with certainty the boundaries of every possible factual scenario. A recent case analyzing the patient-physician relationship has said that such a relationship can be created by a phone call that "affirmatively advises a prospective patient as to a course of treatment" and the patient foreseeably relies on the advice.[6] By analogy, however, it appears that some degree of interaction, even if it is not face-to-face, will trigger the patient-physician relationship and its corresponding duties. Courts have already ruled that telephone contact, for instance, can be used as evidence a physician is examining a patient.[7] The analogy between phone contact and an exchange of information via the Internet appears to be a close one.

If an exchange of information between patient and physician is found to have established the professional patient-physician relationship, then the physician is generally duty-bound to exercise the requisite standard of care and may be civilly liable for a failure to adhere to such a standard. Advice or information given by a provider under the auspices of the patient-physician relationship can justifiably be relied on by the patient—unlike general health care information made available via the Internet. Pursuant to the establishment of a professional relationship, the patient can assume that any advice or information given by the practitioner ceases to be general information (which the user relies on at his or her own risk) and is specific to him or her and safe to act upon.

Medical Records

Most jurisdictions require health care practitioners engaged in rendering care, treatment, or diagnoses to patients to maintain appropriate medical records. In situations where the patient-physician relationship does not exist, the medical record requirement is also nonexistent. Web site sponsors offering health information only need not worry about the creation or retention of medical records. To the extent, however, that a site is interactive and elicits

---

[6] See *Cogswell v Chapman*, 672 NYS 2d 460 (1998); and *Bienz v Central Suffolk Hosp*, 557 NYS 2d 139.
[7] Id at 254. See also footnote 89.

an individual's medical data, the question of whether the professional patient-physician relationship has been established may arise. If so, the practitioner is obligated to maintain a medical record regarding the encounter. Consequently, it is pivotal to determine the nature of the relationship at the outset, as many other duties and obligations are determined by it.

Most state statutes define a medical record in broad terms. It has been defined as including "chart notes, laboratory reports, correspondence, transcribed records, patient questionnaires and any other record concerning the patient's care, diagnosis or treatment,"[8] "records of hospitals, physicians, or other health care providers, addressing an issue of health relevant to the plaintiff's complaint, whether generated before or subsequent to the event giving rise to the claim . . . ,"[9] and "any oral, written, or other transmission in any form or medium of information that: (i) is entered in the record of a patient or recipient; (ii) identifies or can readily be associated with the identity of a patient or recipient; and (iii) relates to the health care of the patient or recipient."[10]

To the extent medical advice or recommendations are given pursuant to establishment of the patient-physician relationship, a practitioner needs to document it as part of the patient's medical record. If the communication is via the Internet, either Web site or e-mail, it is best to document both the inquiry by the patient and the practitioner's response. While the physician's response may not be problematic, recording the patient's inquiry may present significant logistical problems.

With most e-mail systems, the sender's complete name and address are not reflected in the message itself, in either the electronic or printed versions. In the vast majority of instances, a unique e-mail address, consisting of a series of words, letters, or numbers, is used to identify the sender. Even in instances where a person uses an

---

[8] 1997 Ore ALS 635.
[9] Alaska R Civ Proc 72.1.
[10] Md Code Ann Title 4, Subtitle 3, Sec 4-301(1997).

abbreviation of his or her name, such as *dbrown@aol.com*,[11] this address, when viewed by the recipient, may indicate a message from Dave Brown, Debra Brown, Dan Brown, Don Brown, etc. Other addresses, such as *Mary3@aol.com*,[12] may indicate a first name only, with little else to determine the exact identity of the sender. Physicians or physician staff personnel who retrieve or print out the inquiry may be at a loss to correctly file the information in the appropriate patient chart. From an operational perspective, providers receiving e-mail with insufficient sender identification could transmit a reply message seeking full identification. Substantial expenditure of time and effort could be required by this, however, not to mention the accompanying costs related to personnel time.

Certainly the e-mail system, both direct or through a Web site, has the capability to serve as an effective health information communication tool, provided that certain precautions are taken. Patients who routinely and consistently include their full name, social security number, and/or clinic or hospital number can totally or substantially eliminate the logistical barriers to the recording and filing of their information. This presupposes, however, a high degree of patient compliance in including such information. Full identification with social security and patient numbers also highlights the necessity for a strict confidentiality and privacy policy aimed at restricting access to authorized staff.

---

[11] This e-mail address is intended to be purely fictitious; any reference to a real individual or individuals is unintended and coincidental.
[12] This e-mail address is intended to be purely fictitious; any reference to a real individual or individuals is unintended and coincidental.

Section 2

Health Information on the World Wide Web

Accuracy and Timeliness of Information

One of the major obstacles confronting many Internet users is determining which Web sites contain accurate, authoritative, and timely information. Since virtually anyone with access to a computer is capable of launching and maintaining a Web site, users need to exercise great caution before relying too heavily on posted information.

A good starting point for analysis is to investigate the sponsoring organization or individual. In many cases, a site may be maintained by a reputable group or agency in which the user can place great confidence. The federal government has, in many respects, led the way in making health care-related information available on the Internet. Dozens of agency sites, such as those maintained by the US Department of Health & Human Services (HHS), the Health Care Financing Administration (HCFA), and the National Institutes of Health (NIH), regularly post recent developments, proposed and enacted administrative rules, scholarly reports, and other valuable information. Most sites are frequently updated, and in many instances the particular page on which the information is posted displays the date on which the most current update took place.

Accuracy and timeliness of information is a concern to both Web site sponsors and users. The rapidity and frequency of updating will depend, to some extent, on the kind of health information involved. A site purporting to present current health care legislative proposals, for example, may require almost daily modification in order to accurately reflect the pace of legislative activity. By contrast, a site dealing with pharmaceutical approvals by the Food and Drug Administration will probably remain relatively accurate even if it is updated less frequently. The content of Web site information will determine the appropriate degree of frequency.

Authentication and Verification

Because health-related information can be critically important, Web site users should exercise caution in verifying the identity of the Web page sponsor(s). Such reputable Web sites as those maintained by government agencies, health care systems, and private corporations plainly list contact information for their relevant sponsors on the site. Addresses, phone numbers, e-mail addresses, and fax numbers are just some of the information sponsors make available to users. Other sites go further and include rosters or listings of personnel or departments within an organization with whom users can follow up. Contact information of this type permits users not only to verify the accuracy of information but also to inquire further where appropriate.

Many professional organizations, such as medical specialty associations and trade groups, offer valuable information on their Web sites while listing specific contact data. While such information frequently serves primarily as a membership recruitment vehicle, it also doubles as a resource. As a consequence, health care providers planning to sponsor a Web site should carefully consider the way in which contact information is displayed and anticipate questions and concerns users may have.

In general, health care-related information posted on a Web site with little or no information on the sponsor should be viewed with caution. If a sponsoring individual or group is disclosed, the user may be well served by ascertaining what connection, if any, the sponsor has to the Web site content. For instance, a pharmaceutical concern may present clinical data indicating that particular diseases or conditions are appropriately treated by a regime of drug therapy. If the user is aware that the sponsor is a member of the pharmaceutical industry, he or she may next wish to consult other sources or view other Web sites to determine whether other alternatives that may not have been listed are also available. This is not to imply that the sponsor might have any improper motive; rather, depending on the particular experience and expertise of the sponsoring entity, the full spectrum of clinical options simply may not have been presented. From the sponsor's perspective, space on a Web site is limited, requiring a prioritization of information to be included and excluded. Conversely, from the user's perspective, comparing the identity of the sponsor with the scope of content may offer a more accurate picture of the accuracy and comprehensiveness of the information available on a given site.

Interactive Web Sites

At first glance, interactive Web sites do not appear to present significant legal issues. If a health care clinician or organization like a primary care clinic maintains a Web site with clinician information, phone numbers, addresses, etc, there are few legal issues to analyze. When the Web site permits some type of interaction, however, the situation often warrants closer scrutiny.

Interaction can take many different forms: a Web page soliciting such demographics as age and gender to "steer" the user to appropriate information, for instance, or the provision of extensive individual information by the user such as primary complaints, drug allergies, medical history, etc. In the former case, the Web site sponsor's arguable intent is to direct the user to the most relevant and germane cache of information available on its site without making it necessary for the user to browse through information irrelevant to him or her. In the latter, chances are greater the user will see the resultant answers to questions as being specifically applicable to him or her, thereby increasing the chance that the user will more heavily rely on answers received. The intent of the Web site sponsor may be the same in both situations, though the expectations of the user may vary substantially.

With modern technology making so many options available, an increasing number of Web sites offer some degree of interactivity. While such features are very alluring and impressive to users, they are not offered without potential consequence to the Web site sponsor. Depending on the particular facts involved in the dissemination of health information through an interactive site, the following issues can arise:

- whether a professional relationship, such as patient-physician, is created when the site is used,

- whether the sponsoring clinician is properly licensed in all relevant jurisdictions,

- whether adequate steps have been taken to ensure the privacy and confidentiality of transmitted information, and

- whether a disclaimer should be used and, if so, how extensive it should be.

The larger issues just mentioned can also trigger such residual questions as:

- Should a medical record be maintained?

- What information should be included in the medical record, and what should not be considered part of it?
- Is informed consent required and, if so, who bears responsibility for obtaining it?

There is some danger that an interactive Web site providing health information could be construed by the user as the provision of professional medical advice and, thus, imply the patient-physician relationship and its corollary duties. As a general rule, the patient-physician relationship is created through the mutual consent and expectation of the parties. Though it is often construed as a contractual relationship in a legal sense, it need not arise pursuant to a written document. The relationship is most commonly created through conduct that both parties contemplate as encompassing the traditional patient-physician relationship. Office visits, hospitalizations, outpatient procedures, and physicals are just a few of the events that create the patient-physician relationship, even in the absence of a written contract.

Another issue with profound repercussions deals with whether the use of a Web site may subject the provider-sponsor to the jurisdiction of a foreign court, ie, the jurisdiction of the court of a state in which the Web sponsor has no physical presence. Though it appears that the law is still developing in this area, early cases suggest that courts may be swayed by the degree of interactivity offered by the Web site. Though not cases arising from a health environment, 2 recent decisions of federal courts seem to distinguish between "active" and "passive" sites.

In *GTE New Media Services, Inc, v Ameritech Corp*,[13] the court looked at what factors should be considered in determining jurisdiction when a Web site involves some degree of interactivity. Though examined in the context of an antitrust case, the court's opinion

---

[13] 21 F Supp 2d 27 (1998).

offers valuable insight into the factors health care providers may encounter. The *GTE* court looked at 2 factors: the nature of the interaction (eg, commercial aspects) and the quality of the interaction (eg, what level of participation is there via the site). In finding that the court did have jurisdiction over the parties, the court said there was a high level of interaction based on 3 aspects:

1. the defendant actively sought an exchange of information with Web site users,

2. users actively participated by either inputting information or by clicking on an icon, and

3. the Web site linked to other commercial Web sites.

In contrast, courts have viewed passive Web sites in a different light. A case involving trademark rights, *SF Hotel Co v Energy Investments, Inc*, held that a Web site which merely provides general information is insufficient to establish jurisdiction.[14] The plaintiff asserted, in part, that the defendant's Web site activities were enough for the court to secure jurisdiction. The site presented information about the hotel to users and did *not* provide direct communication between the hotel and Web site users.

The opinion of the court thoroughly reviews some of the factors a court evaluates in making jurisdiction determinations. In relevant part, the *SF Hotel* court, citing from *Zippo Mfg Co v Zippo Dot Com, Inc*, said[15]:

> The Internet makes it possible to conduct business throughout the world entirely from a desktop. With this global revolution looming on the horizon, the development of the law concerning the permissible scope of personal jurisdiction based on Internet use is in its infant stages. The cases are

---

[14] 985 F Supp 1032 (1997).
[15] 952 F Supp 1119 (WD Pa 1997).

Using the Internet for Health Information: Legal Issues 17

scant. Nevertheless, our review of the available cases and materials reveals that the likelihood that personal jurisdiction can be constitutionally exercised is directly proportionate to the nature and quality of commercial activity that an entity conducts over the Internet. This sliding scale is consistent with well-developed personal jurisdiction principles. At one end of the spectrum are situations where a defendant clearly does business over the Internet. If the defendant enters into contracts with residents of a foreign jurisdiction that involve the knowing and repeated transmission of computer files over the Internet, personal jurisdiction is proper. E.g. CompuServe, Inc. v. Patterson, 89 F.3d 1257 (6th Cir.1996). At the opposite end are situations where a defendant has simply posted information on an Internet Web site which is accessible to users in foreign jurisdictions. A passive Web site that does little more than make information available to those who are interested in it is not grounds for the exercise of personal jurisdiction. E.g. Bensusan Restaurant Corp. v. King, 937 F. Supp. 295 (S.D.N.Y.1996). The middle ground is occupied by interactive Web sites where a user can exchange information with the host computer. In these cases, the exercise of jurisdiction is determined by examining the level of interactivity and commercial nature of the exchange of information that occurs on the Web site. E.g. Maritz, Inc. v. Cybergold, Inc., 947 F. Supp. 1328 (E.D.Mo.1996).[16]

These cases arguably draw some early distinctions between the mere offering of information to users, on the one hand, and extensive interaction between a health care provider and site user, on

---

[16] 952 F Supp 1119, 1123-24.

the other hand. As this type of electronic exchange of information between providers and patient-users increases, it is likely that courts will continue to be presented with disputes that the parties will turn to the courts to resolve.

State Medical Licensure

Intertwined with the patient-physician relationship is the question of medical licensure. If the degree of Web site listserv or e-mail interactivity is sufficient to create the patient-physician relationship, it then becomes important for the physician to ensure that the patient to whom advice is given resides in the same state in which the physician is medically licensed. Otherwise, the physician may be at risk for illegally practicing medicine in a jurisdiction in which he or she does not hold a license to practice. Although the Internet has existed for many years and the concept of telemedicine continues to evolve and expand, there is currently no statute or judicial decision that has definitively determined whether an Internet "patient" is transported to the physician or the physician transported to the patient. As a result, questions regarding medical licensure remain, and the safest, most conservative approach for a physician wishing to deliver professional advice over the Internet is to be properly licensed in each state in which patients are located.

One of the perils of operating an interactive Web site is making clear to the user the limitations of the site and taking reasonable steps to ensure that the expectations of both the user and site sponsor are the same. A site sponsor intending to share health information or market its services and products needs to evaluate carefully how the site is perceived by users. There is, arguably, a danger that users who reasonably believe the site is offering professional advice may seek to make legal claims against the sponsor should unsatisfactory results occur. To emphasize site limitations, many sites use disclaimers as a vehicle to specify both the intent of the information presented and the limitations the sponsor seeks to impose (disclaimers are discussed in length in a separate segment of this book).

Whenever site interactivity has the potential to affect which information is provided to a user, the risk of user misperception exists. For instance, a site offering standard cardiovascular information may delineate which information is relevant to male populations vs female, and clinical studies may very well justify this. When a user accesses this site, a preliminary prompt asking whether information is sought for males or females or designated age groups (eg, age 35 and below, 36–45, 46–55) may help to direct the user to the appropriate body of information. More extensive interaction, however, such as asking whether specified medical conditions exist (eg, diabetes, hypertension, obesity), may lead the user to believe the information displayed as a result of the prompts is specific to him or her and may therefore reasonably be relied on. The mere display of prepackaged health information, like that in the first example, poses few legal risks to Web site hosts and sponsors. The second example, however, in which several prompts are first answered by the user, increases the danger that a user may see such information as person-specific.

Unfortunately, the analyses of whether interactivity poses a risk are performed on a case-by-case basis. Since no 2 cases are identical, it is likely that courts will be grappling with these issues for quite some time. Further complicating the resolution of these matters will be the continuing development of Internet-related technology, the availability of sophisticated health information, and greater expectations by consumers/users for medical information and data. Just as decades ago health information on the Internet was virtually nonexistent, the decades ahead will likely make current technology and expectations obsolete by comparison.

Section 3

Issues in Health Care Communication via E-mail

Using E-mail to Communicate Health Care Information

As with any communication within the confines of the patient-physician relationship, the privacy and confidentiality of sensitive electronic information is paramount. The use of e-mail to communicate with patients, or for physicians to communicate with each other about patients, does not eliminate the need to ensure confidentiality of sensitive information. Several legal issues are presented by the use of e-mail for the transmission of patient data, including those related to confidentiality and privacy, encryption, patient consent, and medical record retention and storage.

Confidentiality and Privacy of E-mail

In many respects, e-mail is an excellent communication medium for physicians and patients alike. Each can send the other messages that can be retrieved at a time convenient for the recipient. Messages can be sent at any time, 24 hours a day, from virtually anywhere in the world with an Internet connection. Such a capability, however, is not without potential pitfalls.

The use of e-mail can be expected to steadily increase in the years ahead. E-mail use has been reported to have increased from 100,000 users in the late 1970s to approximately 50 million users in 1997.[17] Over 100 million users have been predicted by the year 2000.[18]

Simply stated, the Internet is a network of interconnected computer systems using various Internet service providers (ISPs) to link senders. Throughout the world hundreds of ISPs operate and maintain the infrastructure necessary for the various electronic equipment and communication lines. Such equipment, though normally extremely reliable, is subject to occasional breakdown, malfunction, or interruption. When this occurs, messages may never reach their destination, may become distorted during transmission, or may be misrouted to an unintended recipient. Such situations are of concern whenever they occur, but especially so when the content of the message contains patient-specific medical information that is confidential in nature.

E-mail senders typically have no control over the actual infrastructure used to send messages, unless the transmission is over a dedicated line totally within the domain of the sender. More frequently, multiple ISPs may be employed along the message path. For instance, two ISPs prominent in the United States are America Online (AOL) and MindSpring. A person using AOL as an ISP who sends e-mail to a recipient using MindSpring should be aware that the message, at a minimum, travels through both the AOL and MindSpring infrastructures. Somewhere along this message routing, errors may occur, causing the message to be misrouted—sent to an unintended recipient. A misdirected medical message is extremely problematic, as breaches in confidentiality may occur.

Knowing that such malfunctions sometimes occur, senders of confidential information should do whatever they can to minimize such dangers.

---

[17] Kane B, Sands DZ. Guidelines for the clinical use of electronic mail with patients [white paper]. *JAMIA* [serial online]. January-February 1998;5. Available at: http://www.amia.org/positio1.htm. Accessed April 13, 1999.

[18] Id.

E-mail Between Patients and Providers

Health care providers are finding it increasingly attractive to communicate with patients through e-mail. E-mail's many advantages offer convenience to physician and patient alike: Messages can be sent at any time of the day or night without inconveniencing the recipient; messages can be read at any time convenient for the recipient; costs of transmission are minimal; printouts of messages can be retained when desired; and messages can be sent or retrieved from virtually any location with Internet access. As important as these advantages are, using the Internet for this purpose is not without potential drawbacks—some very substantial. Reputable organizations have already drafted guidelines addressing many of the critical areas of concern involving the use of e-mail for health care information.[19]

Privacy and confidentiality of message content is again a critical concern. Consider the following scenarios, all of which create serious privacy and confidentiality breaches:

- The sending practitioner mistakenly inserts the wrong address, perhaps only missing one keyboard character of information.

- Despite a correct address, technical problems with the Internet service provider misroute the address to an unintended recipient.

- The recipient's e-mail is read by someone else with access to the e-mail account: parent, spouse, or child at home, or a colleague at work.

These scenarios can occur with either party acting as the message receiver. Just as there is a danger that family members may inadvertently access information intended for a patient, it must be remembered that errors can also occur when the physician is the

---

[19] Kane B, Sands DZ. Guidelines for the clinical use of electronic mail with patients [white paper]. *JAMIA* [serial online]. January-February 1998;5. Available at: http://www.amia.org/positio1.htm. Accessed April 13, 1999.

intended recipient. A physician accessing e-mail at home may risk his or her family member mistakenly viewing patient messages, or an unauthorized clerk in the practitioner's office may have access. The combinations are almost endless.

To minimize errors associated with the use of e-mail between patients and health care providers, consideration should be given to the use of an e-mail agreement, a mutual understanding between the parties intending to use e-mail to communicate with each other. Providers and patients who enter into such an agreement can spell out with specificity the limits imposed on e-mail communication of health information. By way of example and not limitation, the following areas may be addressed in a patient-provider e-mail agreement.

Content
Agreement on what kind of health care information is acceptable for inclusion in an e-mail message is important. The parties may agree that simple health care questions, requests and orders for prescriptions, requests and scheduling of office appointments, disclosure of test results, and medical reminders may be appropriate. On the other hand, the parties may forbid the transmission of highly sensitive information such as mental health records, HIV status, and medical information related to such pending legal claims or litigation as a medical malpractice or workers' compensation claim. Inquiries of an emergency nature should be avoided, and patients should be advised not to rely on e-mail communication in such situations.

Identity of Message Readers
In an effort to preserve the highest degree of patient confidentiality and privacy, the parties' disclosure of who will be reading e-mail messages is crucial. The provider should disclose whether mail will always be read by him or her personally, and the patient should

reveal whether only he or she will be able to access the message or, conversely, whether other family members or friends may be able to read messages on occasion. Additionally, the provider may disclose that his or her nurse will be reading e-mail messages, or that any nurse in the office might have access to e-mails. In the former case, the patient may have confidence and comfort, but the latter may not be acceptable, depending on the size of the office and the number of personnel involved. Providers using aides, secretaries, etc, to process e-mail may find it especially important to disclose this in advance to patients to ensure that they do not object.

Response Time

To reduce unreasonable expectations and potential confusion between the parties, providers and patients should agree on the response time expected of each party. Each should disclose how frequently they retrieve and read e-mail and how quickly they will generally respond to inquiries. Differences in expected response time for weekdays and weekends should also be addressed. In addition, providers may wish to advise patients of differentials in typical response times, depending on the nature of the inquiry. Confirmation of an upcoming office appointment may, for instance, allow a longer response time than an inquiry about a prescription dosage or a complaint about possible medication side effects.

Use and Retention of Messages

Whenever possible, electronic and/or paper copies of patient e-mails and corresponding responses should be retained by the provider as parts of the patient's medical record. To facilitate this, patients should be asked to clearly state their full name, clinic number, patient identification, etc, in messages so that proper record-keeping can be achieved. Furthermore, patients should be advised that message content should be focused on factual matters and unnecessary gossip avoided.

Overriding E-mail With Personal Calls

For the benefit of patient and provider alike, the parties should reach a common understanding on what to do if the reason for an e-mail message escalates into a more serious matter while the patient awaits a response. Patients should know when to phone the provider, page him or her, or proceed to an urgent care clinic or emergency room when the situation warrants.

Encryption

The use of passwords and encryption can benefit both providers and patients. In an effort to clarify the expectations of both parties, some type of patient-provider e-mail agreement should be used and the subject of e-mail privacy technology addressed in the document. For instance, it would be helpful to state the software or encryption technology the parties have agreed to use or, conversely, that the parties agree not to use such options. A mutual understanding between patient and provider is essential to effective e-mail communication and the prevention of false expectations.

Incorporating E-mail Technology

An important part of preserving patient confidentiality and privacy in e-mail transmissions is the use of encryption technology as discussed in this section. Since the user friendliness, cost, and availability of such technology will likely continue to change in coming years, health care providers should carefully monitor new developments and incorporate enhanced technology whenever possible.

Mailing Lists and Newsgroups

The mass distribution of e-mail correspondence to members of designated groups with an interest in a common topic like health care is increasing. Electronic mailing lists automatically direct all messages sent to their main address to all members of the list."[20] Mailing lists permit persons who wish to communicate with others with similar interests via the Internet to easily do so by "subscribing" to lists. Usually the subscription is free and entails e-mails sent by individual list members to be shared with other subscribers. Often, members may pose questions, hoping that other members may share helpful information or even offer specific answers to their inquiries. Lists address almost every topic imaginable, from electronics to mechanics to gardening to health care.

Similar to lists, newsgroups are the Internet version of a bulletin board. On newsgroups, people can post and reply to public messages on particular topics.[21] Generally considered to be broader in scope than lists, newsgroups offer yet another opportunity for those with common interests to exchange ideas and information. Messages posted to newsgroups can be read by anyone with access to the group, and anyone may choose to respond to a posting. Like lists, newsgroups focus on virtually every topic one can imagine, including hundreds specifically relating to health care and medicine. Newsgroups are so numerous that one Internet service provider, MindSpring, offers its users over 20,000 newsgroups to choose from.[22] At last estimate, there were over 80,000 active newsgroups available through the Internet.

The use of lists and newsgroups for health care generates perplexing legal questions. As with typical health care–related information, concerns relating to confidentiality, privacy, licensure, and the patient-physician relationship arise. Most lists and newsgroup users are aware that their postings (ie, messages or e-mails) are not confidential to any degree and are shared with the list members. Consequently, they post confidential information about themselves or others at their own peril and do not expect any type of privacy or confidentiality. Sometimes, however, postings in a health care area may describe a particular condition or malady and

---

[20] Goldman N. Glossary. *The Complete Idiot's Pocket Reference to the Internet.* Indianapolis, Ind: Alpha Books; 1994:204.
[21] Goldman N. Glossary. *The Complete Idiot's Pocket Reference to the Internet.* Indianapolis, Ind: Alpha Books; 1994:205.
[22] Search of MindSpring newsgroups. Available at: www.mindspring.net. Accessed January 12, 1999.

seek recommendations on a future course of treatment or possible diagnoses. Response postings with specific recommendations carry the risk of being perceived as authoritative, reliable, and specific to the original inquiry. Such a scenario creates the danger that a list or newsgroup recipient may interpret the response as the equivalent of professional medical advice and rely on it, notwithstanding the intent of the sender that it be nothing more than a sharing of general information.

It is in this way that the issues of licensure and the patient-physician relationship emerge. Physicians are licensed to practice medicine by the individual states in which they practice. There is no national medical license enabling physicians to practice in any state, or all states, without obtaining individual state licensure or qualifying for statutory licensure exceptions, exclusions, or exemptions.

The medical practice acts of most states define the "practice of medicine" to include providing medical advice, rendering a diagnosis, developing a treatment plan, prescribing medications, and conducting diagnostics on patients. For instance, in relevant part, Alabama defines the practice of medicine to include: "diagnose, treat, correct, advise or prescribe for any human disease, ailment, injury, infirmity, deformity, pain or other condition, physical or mental, real or imaginary, by any means or instrumentality."[23] Similarly, Kentucky defines its practice of medicine to include: "the diagnosis, treatment, or correction of any and all human conditions, ailments, diseases, injuries, or infirmities by any and all means, methods, devices, or instrumentalities."[24] Many such statutes, by virtue of their terminology, are broad in their application.

Health care practitioners need to carefully review the role they play in lists and newsgroups to avoid the appearance of creating a professional relationship or the rendering of medical advice with-

---

[23] Michie's Alabama Code §34-24-50 (1998).
[24] KRS §311.550 (Michie 1998).

in the parameters of the patient-physician relationship. Some lists include a brief disclaimer in each message as a way of reinforcing the limitations of the information set forth. The American Health Lawyers Association (AHLA) incorporates the following notice in its list's messages: "Postings to this list are not confidential. The information obtained by the use of this service is for reference use only and does not constitute the rendering of legal, financial, or other professional advice by American Health Lawyers Association" (J. Salerno [jsalerno@healthlawyers.org], e-mail, April 15, 1999). Apart from tailoring the content of messages, the use of such notices in lists and newsgroups can be helpful in framing the extent to which information should be relied on.

Section 4
Strategies for Cyberspace Risk Management

Encryption

One mechanism to minimize the risk of messages being read by unintended recipients, whether via misrouting, equipment malfunction, or unanticipated persons accessing the receiving computer, is to employ encryption technology. Encryption is defined as a method of storing data so that it is accessible only to those with the requisite password and lets a reader restrict who has access to his or her messages.[25] Unauthorized readers who have not been given the requisite password are prevented from gaining message access.

Practitioners transmitting identifiable patient health care data or information, such as diagnoses, treatment plans, x-ray images, etc, should consider incorporating available encryption technology as a way to maintain confidentiality. The Health Care Financing Administration (HCFA) has already issued guidelines regarding the type of information that can be sent via the Internet.[26] Using encryption can address many potential confidentiality issues, including:

- reading of messages by unintended recipients caused by message misrouting due to equipment malfunctions,

---

[25] Goldman N. Glossary. *The Complete Idiot's Pocket Reference to the Internet.* Indianapolis, Ind: Alpha Books; 1994:203.
[26] See Appendix B, HCFA Internet Security Policy, issued November 24, 1998.

31

- reading of messages by others in the recipient's office who are unauthorized for the patient or case in question,
- offering greater assurances to the message sender that accidental breaches will not occur, and
- being able to trace breaches to those provided the requisite password.

Possible economic savings have sometimes prompted physicians maintaining multiple offices to consider conveying information via Internet e-mail in lieu of using couriers to ferry messages and x-rays from one location to another. While lower costs and increased convenience may justify such a transition, any decision should include a risk analysis for possible confidentiality breaches. Depending on the computer systems involved and the technology employed, encryption may provide a suitable alternative.

Once encryption is used, health care practitioners should periodically examine the marketplace to check for new and improved encryption alternatives. Utilizing then state-of-the-art encryption technology does not guarantee such technology will forever be appropriate or meet the professional standard expected of health care practitioners. Vigilance of the encryption market is advised.

Malpractice Insurance

In the event the patient-physician relationship is established over the Internet, physicians need to be mindful of the scope and limitations of their medical malpractice insurance. Many policies provide insurance for specified individuals at designated locations. Frequently, malpractice insurance applications will require the applicant to set forth the location or locations of the medical practice in order to be insured. This provides full disclosure to the insurer and affords the company's underwriters an opportunity to assess the risk associated with the jurisdiction involved. Medical malpractice underwriters may determine that the risks of practicing in state 1 are different than in state 2 due, in part, to differences in:

- statutes of limitations,
- rules of procedure and rules of evidence,
- existence or absence of medical malpractice damage caps, and
- the scope of medical practice acts.

Additionally, insurers normally are required to be licensed to offer insurance in each state in which they conduct business. Covering a malpractice claim for an incident in a jurisdiction that was not previously disclosed may present a serious problem for the insurer. Insurers, therefore, should be advised about the practice-related activities in which physicians are engaged, including the use or sponsorship of Web sites, e-mail, Internet discussion groups, mailing lists, etc.

Communication with the medical malpractice insurer is critical. Initial applicants for malpractice insurance should be careful to disclose the full scope of their professional activities, including those that are Internet and e-mail related. Physicians who desire to expand their practice through the use of a Web site, telemedicine, or e-mail (when such activities were not previously used or disclosed) should also contact their insurer even if they are midway into the policy term. Clarification that coverage for Internet and e-mail activities exists should also be secured in situations where the policy language is ambiguous or where it appears that policy exclusions may include the desired activity. The optimal time for clarification, of course, is before the activity is undertaken and while the policyholder physician is still in a position to negotiate with the insurer over the additional coverage, if necessary.

Malpractice insurers may also have prerequisites to, or recommendations for, risk management initiatives to pursue in using the Internet, Web sites, or e-mail. As technology continues to evolve and Internet use spirals, insurers will likely become more active in developing policies to deal with Internet- and telemedicine-related issues.

At a conference in Washington, DC, in September 1998, a representative of the Physician Insurers Association of America (PIAA) addressed several measures physician providers may consider implementing regarding the use of the Internet for transmission of health care information. Among measures to be considered were:

- the use of encryption for transmittal of patient records;
- requesting, whenever possible, confirmation from the recipient that information was properly received; this can be especially important when transmitting patient-specific data between health care providers;
- providers sponsoring Web sites using peer-reviewed material as resources for patients and Web site users;
- exercising caution in determining whether, and with whom, to link to other Web sites;
- keeping information current and up-to-date if a Web site is to be used; and
- providers using the Internet to communicate with patients or other providers developing policies governing access to e-mail messages. Staff computer access should be limited to business purposes only, access should be restricted by passwords, and all patient e-mail messages should be retained.[27]

---

[27] Bartholomew L. In Legal environment of telemedicine, presentation of the Physician Insurers Association of America; September 28, 1999; Washington, DC.

Rationales for Disclaimers

Disclaimers are important for several reasons. In practical terms, they can articulate for the viewer the scope of information available and any restrictions or limitations associated with it. The restriction may be as simple as an acknowledgment that currency of materials is not guaranteed, thus prompting the user to verify the accuracy of information before relying on it. Or a disclaimer may include a warning that, despite some degree of interaction, a professional patient-physician relationship is not created and the information received is not to be construed as the practice of medicine. While both types of disclaimer are important, their geneses are different. The former highlights information limitations, while the latter is required due to concerns over practitioner licensure, medical malpractice insurance coverage, etc.

The Internet is an especially logical place to use disclaimers because there is no face-to-face contact with the user, and the site sponsor usually has no way of determining the jurisdiction (ie, state or country) in which the user resides. The residence of the user can also present a significant obstacle to a provider dispensing information via the Internet.

If the provider is a physician, nurse, pharmacist, or other professional required to hold a license to practice medicine, the provision of information over the Internet to a person of an unknown residence can be dangerous. Several questions arise. What if the information provided by the physician or other professional can be construed as the "practice" of medicine or the dispensing of professional advice? If the user resides in a state other than the one in which the provider is licensed, is the provider at risk for unlawfully practicing in a jurisdiction without the requisite license? The provider using the Internet to communicate with patients, then, has several reasons to be concerned about properly establishing the nature and boundaries of the relationship.

The difference between sharing information and rendering advice may be subtle, but the ramifications of such a distinction are great. One may require a medical license, while the other may not. One may expose the provider to malpractice concerns, while the other may not. One of the easiest ways of attempting to deal with such concerns is through the use of disclaimers aimed at defining the nature of the relationship.

By advancing the disclaimer to the user upon arrival at the site, the sponsor informs the user about the nature of the site and lets the user recognize and agree to the "ground rules." If nothing else, this action arguably assists in deflecting unreasonable expectations that the user might have had without any such notification. The legal validity of disclaimers, however, is not guaranteed. Should a dispute arise over the applicability or enforceability of a disclaimer, courts would look to the specific facts and circumstances present in a legal case. Since no 2 cases are identical, it is virtually impossible to articulate universally acceptable rules in using disclaimers on the Internet.

The Use of Disclaimers in Health Care Web Sites

As the availability of health information via the Internet continues to proliferate, Web site sponsors and health care providers are increasingly using disclaimers as a means to define the limitations of the information offered. Disclaimers have long been used in the law, particularly in contractual matters when the parties seek to memorialize their understandings. A disclaimer is defined as:

> The repudiation or renunciation of a claim or power vested in a person or which he had formerly alleged to be his. The refusal, or rejection of an estate or right offered to a person. The disavowal, denial, or renunciation of an interest, right, or property imputed to a person or alleged to be his. Also the declaration, or the instrument, by which such disclaimer is published.[28]

Many Web sites offering health care information (either through access to journals, articles, and studies, or by user interaction that elicits a response from a health care provider) employ disclaimers to define the relationship between the site and the user. The posting of a disclaimer on a Web site can be handled in a variety of ways. The disclaimer can be represented by a "button" marked as a disclaimer and always available to the user any time he or she wishes, or it can be the first screen presented to the viewer upon accessing the site. Another variation is the presentation of the disclaimer immediately upon accessing the site with 2 buttons the user can choose from at the end of the document. One indicates the user has read and agrees to the terms and conditions specified in the disclaimer, while the other denotes the user does not agree. In cases where the user does not agree, further access to the site is denied or access is restricted to other areas.

The particular variation of disclaimer to use will likely depend on the nature of information offered via the Web site, its clinical significance, and the role the site is intended to play between provider and user. For sites offering information on general health topics, a disclaimer that is always available for the user to read may be sufficient, even if the patient/user ignores it. Web sites containing more clinically significant content may require the user to acknowledge that he or she has *both* read the disclaimer and agreed to its terms before being permitted to access additional information.

---

[28] Black HC et al, eds. *Black's Law Dictionary.* Rev 4th ed. St Paul, Minn: West Publishing Co; 1968:550.

A relatively new service called *America's Doctor* (URL: www.americasdoctor.com) offers Internet users an on-line opportunity to "chat" with a physician about particular health conditions or topics. The user is able to log on to the site and interact with a physician through an exchange of messages. While no fee is charged, the site requires that a user agree to specific terms and limitations before the exchange with a provider takes place. The disclaimer is very thorough and addresses several important aspects, including the following.

- The site should not be used for emergencies.

- Agreement that any controversies arising from use of the site will be resolved in accordance with the laws of a particular state. (In this case, Maryland is designated.)

- Persons pursuing legal action arising from use of the service agree to waive their right to a jury trial.

- The user is at least 18 years old.

- No patient-physician relationship is created by use of the service, and information given by providers does not constitute the practice of medicine.

- Additionally, the information secured from the site is not to be construed as a substitute for a professional relationship with a physician.

- No professional relationships are established by interaction with nurses or pharmacists.

- *America's Doctor* will not retain any medical records in connection with the physician-consumer "chat" encounter.

- There will be no monitoring of the user's care.

- *America's Doctor* will neither take payment from nor bill any party.[29]

---

[29] America's Doctor. Disclaimer. Available at: http://www.americasdoctor.com. Accessed April 13, 1999.

On this particular Web site, agreeing with the disclaimer is mandatory. Those selecting the button that reflects that they do not agree will not be able to interact with a provider. A user who thoroughly and thoughtfully reads the disclaimer will likely have a much clearer understanding of the limitations envisioned by *America's Doctor*. Understanding the disclaimer before using the service will also greatly reduce the user's likelihood of confusion later.

Another method of using a disclaimer on a health care-related Web site is employed by the Mayo Clinic. At its site,[30] the Mayo Clinic lists, in small print at the bottom of the page, "Legal Restrictions and Terms of Use Applicable To This Site."[31] The site language also includes: "use of this site signifies your agreement to the terms of use."[32] The intent is to notify the user that if he or she proceeds with using the site, it is implied that he or she agrees to the terms outlined in the disclaimer.

There also are Web sites that permit patients to interact with providers for a fee. In such instances, provider licensing issues become even more important, and the provider's ability to verify the location of the user is paramount. For instance, psychotherapy services via the Internet give users the ability to ask short questions of a provider in exchange for a fee.[33] Licensure in these cases becomes very important, depending on the scope and breadth of the applicable licensing statute.

Some site sponsors may wish to retain an electronic copy of the user's acquiescence to the disclaimer for possible use as a defense in the event a dispute arises. Though this will not be as effective as a signed contract with the user, it arguably can be used as a mechanism by which to identify the user through their computer identification.

---

[30] See http://www.mayohealth.org/mayo/common/htm/disclaim.
[31] See http://www.mayohealth.org. See also Appendix D.
[32] Id.
[33] Pergament D. Internet psychotherapy: current status and future regulation [note]. *Health Matrix*. Summer 1998;8:247.

As the volume and sophistication of health information on the Internet continue to increase, the number of on-line providers will also rise. Over time, disputes that are taken to the courts for resolution will offer additional insight into the effectiveness and validity of disclaimers and similar notices. Just as the computer technology industry is not static, so too is the law fluid as it relates to this relatively new medium.

The E-mail Agreement

An agreement between a health care provider and patient regarding the use of e-mail can be established in a number of ways. A simple memorandum or letter outlining issues that have been discussed and signed by the patient can be very effective. Though oral agreements may suffice in some situations, a written document can refresh a patient's memory as to what has been agreed to. Additionally, in instances where the provider and patient have differing recollections, a written memo can set the record straight. A more formal document listing the permissible uses of e-mail for dissemination of health care information, message response time, technology used (or waiver of liability for nonuse), and an indemnity or hold-harmless clause for technical problems generally considered to be beyond the control of the provider or user may also be used as a means of recording the understanding between the parties. The scope of an e-mail agreement could include the following:

- designation of authorized users (ie, specify patient, providers, and the e-mail address of each);
- use of special encryption technology and, if used, what kind (in the event the parties opt not to use encryption, a waiver indicating the voluntary omission of such technology should be included);

- the permissible scope of content to be used in e-mail and specific exclusions for information that is *not* to be sent via e-mail;
- the response time agreed to by the parties;
- a statement that certain conditions may warrant the patient ignore e-mail and call the physician, use an urgent care clinic, or proceed to an emergency room;
- a hold-harmless and indemnity provision protecting parties from liability for technical problems beyond their control (eg, power outages, system failures by an Internet service provider);
- the type of identifying information to be included in patient e-mail (eg, full name, social security number, hospital patient number, clinic number); and
- recitation that hard copies of e-mail messages will be retained as a part of the patient's medical record.

Conclusion

There should be little doubt regarding the size, popularity, and utility of the Internet and e-mail as means of communicating with health care providers and retrieving valuable health information. This is true both within the United States and globally. The knowledge level of patient-consumers—and their expectations—will undoubtedly grow in the years ahead. As a consequence, the Internet will become an increasingly useful tool for exchanging health information.

The convenience and popularity of Internet technology should not, however, erase concerns regarding the legal issues associated with the electronic transmission of health information. Privacy, confidentiality, medical record creation and maintenance, malpractice insurance coverage, provider licensure, and the Internet's relationship with health information will remain important as legal issues involving electronic medicine develop. Careful monitoring of legal developments in the years ahead will result in considerable benefit in evaluating the intersection of medicine and the Internet. The ultimate goal should be using Internet and e-mail technologies to assist everyone involved in the rendition of health care—patients, providers, institutions, and third-party payers—without jeopardizing the integrity, accuracy, or confidentiality of such information. As technology advances, those involved in health care will need to keep abreast of statutory changes and judicial opinions bearing upon how such technology can be appropriately used for health care purposes.

Appendix A

Warning to Internet Users From Minnesota Attorney General

WARNING TO ALL INTERNET USERS AND PROVIDERS

THIS MEMORANDUM SETS FORTH THE ENFORCEMENT POSITION OF THE MINNESOTA ATTORNEY GENERAL'S OFFICE WITH RESPECT TO CERTAIN ILLEGAL ACTIVITIES ON THE INTERNET.

PERSONS OUTSIDE OF MINNESOTA WHO TRANSMIT INFORMATION VIA THE INTERNET KNOWING THAT INFORMATION WILL BE DISSEMINATED IN MINNESOTA ARE SUBJECT TO JURISDICTION IN MINNESOTA COURTS FOR VIOLATIONS OF STATE CRIMINAL AND CIVIL LAWS.

The following discussion sets out the legal basis for this conclusion.

Minnesota's general criminal jurisdiction statute provides as follows:

Source: Minnesota Attorney General's Office. Warning to Internet users from Minnesota Attorney General. Available at:
http://www.webcom.com/~lewrose/article/minn.html.
Accessed April 1, 1999.

A person may be convicted and sentenced under the law of this State if the person:

> (1) Commits an offense in whole or in part within this state; or
> (2) Being without the state, causes, aids or abets another to commit a crime within the state; or
> (3) Being without the state, intentionally causes a result within the state prohibited by the criminal laws of this state.
>
> It is not a defense that the defendant's conduct is also a criminal offense under the laws of another state or of the United States or of another country. Minnesota Statute Section 609.025 (1994).

This statute has been interpreted by the Minnesota Supreme Court. In State v. Rossbach, 288 N.W.2d 714 (Minn. 1980), the defendant appealed his conviction for aggravated assault. The defendant, standing inside the border of an Indian Reservation, had fired a rifle across the boundary line at a person outside the border. The defendant claimed that Minnesota courts did not have jurisdiction because his act took place off of Minnesota lands. Applying Minnesota Statute Section 609.025 and the common law, the Minnesota Supreme Court affirmed the conviction, holding that the intentional impact within Minnesota land created jurisdiction. Id. at 715-16.

The Minnesota Court of Appeals reached a similar result in State v. Brown, 486 N.W.2d 816 (Minn. Ct. App. 1992). In Brown, the court implicitly found that Minnesota courts had criminal jurisdiction over individuals in Iowa who mailed unlicensed gambling equipment to Minnesota residents. Id. at 817-18.

Minnesota courts have applied similar jurisdictional principles in civil cases. In State v. Red Lake DFL Committee, 303 N.W.2d 54 (Minn. 1981), the Minnesota Supreme Court held that state courts had jurisdiction over a committee of the Red Lake Indian Tribe which had purchased space for political advertisements in a newspaper circulated in the state. At issue was whether the committee had to register under state ethical practices laws.

The committee argued that it had done nothing outside of the reservation, since the transaction with the newspaper took place inside the reservation, and the committee did not assist in the circulation of the newspaper. In holding that the committee was required to register under state ethical practices law, the Supreme Court responded to this argument as follows:

> Defendants say nothing they did occurred outside the reservation, but they choose to ignore that what they did caused something to occur beyond the reservation boundaries, namely, the dissemination of a political message, which is the activity here sought to be regulated. Id. at 56 (emphasis added [sic]).

The above principles of Minnesota law apply equally to activities on the Internet. Individuals and organizations outside of Minnesota who disseminate information in Minnesota via the Internet and thereby cause a result to occur in Minnesota are subject to state criminal and civil laws.

An Example of Illegal Activity on the Internet—Gambling

Gambling appears to be an especially prominent aspect of criminal activity on the Internet. There are a number of services outside of Minnesota that offer Minnesota residents the opportunity to place bets on sporting events, purchase lottery tickets, and participate in simulated casino games. These services are illegal in Minnesota.

Lotteries

A lottery is defined as "a plan which provides for the distribution of money, property or other reward or benefit to persons selected by chance from among participants some or all of whom have given a consideration for the chance of being selected." Minnesota Statute Section 609.75, Subdivision 1(a)(1994).

Generally, it is unlawful in Minnesota to sell or transfer a chance to participate in a lottery. Minnesota Statute Section 609.755(2) (1994). It is also unlawful to disseminate information in Minnesota about a lottery, except a lottery conducted by an adjoining state, with intent to encourage participation therein. Minnesota Statute Section 609.755(3). Acts in Minnesota in furtherance of a lottery conducted outside of Minnesota are included, notwithstanding its validity where conducted. Minnesota Statute Section 609.75, Subdivision 1(c)(1994). Violation of these provisions is a misdemeanor, punishable by up to 90 days in jail, or a fine of up to $700, or both. Minnesota Statute Section 609.755 (1994); 609.02, Subdivision 3 (1994). It is a gross misdemeanor under Minnesota law to conduct a lottery. Minnesota Statute Section 609.76, Subdivision 1(3) (1994). A gross misdemeanor is punishable by up to one year in jail, or a $3,000 fine, or both. Minnesota Statute Section 609.02, Subdivision 4 (1994).

Sports Bookmaking

Sports bookmaking is defined as "the activity of intentionally receiving, recording or forwarding within any 30-day period more than five bets, or offers to bet, that total more than $2,500 on any one or more sporting events." Minnesota Statute Section 609.75, Subdivision 7 (1994). Engaging in sports bookmaking is a felony, which is punishable by more than one year imprisonment. Minnesota Statutes Sections 609.76, Subdivision 2 (1994); 609.02, Subdivision 2 (1994). Intentionally receiving, recording, or forwarding bets or offers to bet in lesser amounts is a gross misdemeanor. Minnesota Statute Section 609.76, Subdivision 1 (7) (1994).

Accomplice Liability

Minnesota's accomplice statute provides that one who intentionally aids, advises, counsels, or conspires with another to commit a crime is equally liable for that crime. Minnesota Statute Section 609.05, Subdivision 1 (1994). Therefore, persons or organizations who knowingly assist Internet gambling organizations in any unlawful activity may themselves be held liable for that unlawful activity. Thus, for example, Internet access providers and credit card companies that continue to provide services to gambling organizations after notice that the activities of the organizations are illegal would be subject to accomplice liability.

In addition to being illegal under Minnesota law, the Internet gambling organizations appear to violate several provisions of the federal law. All of the services appear to violate 18 United States Code Section 1084, which prohibits the foreign or interstate transmission of bets or wagers or information on bets or wagers by use of a wire communication. In as much as the Internet gambling organizations involve lotteries, they would also appear to violate 18 United States Code Section 1301 (prohibiting the "importing or transporting" of lottery tickets; 18 United States Code Section 1302 (prohibiting the mailing of lottery tickets); and 18 United States Code Section 1304 (prohibiting the "broadcasting" of lottery information). Sections 1084 and 1301 provide for felony-level penalties, while Sections 1302 and 1304 provide for misdemeanor penalties.

Placing a Bet Through Internet Gambling Organizations

Minnesota residents should be aware that it is unlawful to make a bet through Internet gambling organizations. Minnesota law makes it a misdemeanor to place a bet unless done pursuant to an exempted, state-regulated activity, such as licensed charitable gambling or the state lottery. Minnesota Statute Sections 609.75, Subdivisions 2 - 3; 609.755(1) (1994). The Internet gambling organizations are not exempted. Therefore, any person in Minnesota who places a bet through one of these organizations is committing a crime.

Minnesota residents should also be aware of forfeiture provisions related to unlawful gambling activity. Minnesota Statute Section 609.762, Subdivision 1 (1994) provides that the following items are subject to forfeiture:

> (a) Devices used or intended for use, including those defined in Section 349.30, Subdivision 2, as a gambling device, except as authorized in Sections 349.11 to 349.23 and 349.40;
> (b) All moneys, materials, and other property used or intended for use as payment to participate in gambling or a prize or receipt for gambling; and
> (c) Books, records, and research products and materials, including formulas, microfilm, tapes, and data used or intended for use in gambling.

A "gambling device" is defined as "a contrivance which for a consideration affords the player an opportunity to obtain something of value, other than free plays, automatically from the machine or otherwise, the award of which is determined principally by chance." Minnesota Statute Section 609.75, Subdivision 4 (1994).

Under this definition of "gambling device," a computer that is used to play a game of chance for something of value would be subject to forfeiture.

Gambling is just one example of illegal activity on the Internet. However, the same jurisdictional principles apply with equal force to any illegal activity.

Please direct any inquiries regarding this notice, or report violations of Minnesota law to the Law Enforcement Section, Minnesota Attorney General's Office, Suite 1400, NCL Tower, 445 Minnesota Street, St. Paul, Minnesota 55101-2131, telephone 612 296-7575.

Appendix B

HCFA Internet Security Policy

1. Purpose

This bulletin formalizes the policy and guidelines for the security and appropriate use of the Internet to transmit HCFA Privacy Act-protected and other sensitive HCFA information.

2. Effective Date

This bulletin is effective as of the date of issuance.

3. Expiration Date

This bulletin remains in effect until superseded or canceled.

4. Introduction

The Internet is the fastest growing telecommunications medium in our history. This growth and the easy access it affords has significantly enhanced the opportunity to use advanced information technology for both the public and private sectors. It provides unprecedented opportunities for interaction and data sharing among health care providers,

---

Source: Health Care Financing Administration. HCFA Internet security policy. November 24, 1998. Available at: http://www.hcfa.gov/security/isecplcy/htm. Accessed April 13, 1999.

HCFA contractors, HCFA components, State agencies acting as HCFA agents, Medicare and Medicaid beneficiaries, and researchers. However, the advantages provided by the Internet come with a significantly greater element of risk to the confidentiality and integrity of information. The very nature of the Internet communication mechanisms means that security risks cannot be totally eliminated. Up to now, because of these security risks and the need to research security requirements vis-à-vis the Internet, HCFA has prohibited the use of the Internet for the transmission of all HCFA Privacy Act-protected and other sensitive HCFA information by its components and Medicare/Medicaid partners, as well as other entities authorized to use this data.

The Privacy Act of 1974 mandates that federal information systems must protect the confidentiality of individually-identifiable data. Section 5 U.S.C. 552a (e) (10) of the Act is very clear; federal systems must: ". . .establish appropriate administrative, technical, and physical safeguards to insure the security and confidentiality of records and to protect against any anticipated threats or hazards to their security or integrity which could result in substantial harm, embarrassment, inconvenience, or unfairness to any individual on whom information is maintained." One of HCFA's primary responsibilities is to assure the security of the Privacy Act-protected and other sensitive information it collects, produces, and disseminates in the course of conducting its operations. HCFA views this responsibility as a covenant with its beneficiaries, personnel, and health care providers. This responsibility is also assumed by HCFA's contractors, State agencies acting as HCFA agents, other government organizations, as well as any entity that has been authorized access to HCFA information resources as a party to a Data Release Agreement with HCFA.

However, HCFA is also aware that there is a growing demand for use of the Internet for inexpensive transmission of Privacy Act-protected and other sensitive information. HCFA has a responsibility to accommodate this desire as long as it can be assured that proper steps are being taken to maintain an acceptable level of security for the information involved.

This issuance is intended to establish the basic security requirements that must be addressed for use of the Internet to transmit HCFA Privacy Act-protected and/or other sensitive HCFA information.

The term "HCFA Privacy Act-protected Data and other sensitive HCFA information" is used throughout this document. This phrase refers to data which, if disclosed, could result in harm to the agency or individual persons. Examples include:

- All individually identifiable data held in systems of records. Also included are automated systems of records subject to the Privacy Act, which contain information that meets the qualifications for Exemption 6 of the Freedom of Information Act; i.e., for which unauthorized disclosure would constitute a "clearly unwarranted invasion of personal privacy" likely to lead to specific detrimental consequences for the individual in terms of financial, employment, medical, psychological, or social standing.

- Payment information that is used to authorize or make cash payments to individuals or organizations. These data are usually stored in production application files and systems, and include benefits information, such as that found at the Social Security Administration (SSA), and payroll information. Such information also includes databases that the user has the authority and capability to use and/or alter. As modification of such records could cause an improper payment, these records must be adequately protected.

- Proprietary information that has value in and of itself and which must be protected from unauthorized disclosure.

- Computerized correspondence and documents that are considered highly sensitive and/or critical to an organization and which must be protected from unauthorized alteration and/or premature disclosure.

5. Policy

This Guide establishes the fundamental rules and systems security requirements for the use of the Internet to transmit HCFA Privacy Act-protected and other sensitive HCFA information collected, maintained, and disseminated by HCFA, its contractors, and agents. It is permissible to use the Internet for transmission of HCFA Privacy Act-protected and/or other sensitive HCFA information, as long as an acceptable method of encryption is utilized to provide for confidentiality and integrity of this data, and that authentication or identification procedures are employed to assure that both the sender and recipient of the data are known to each other and are authorized to receive and decrypt such information. Detailed guidance is provided below in item 7.

6. Scope

This policy covers all systems or processes which use the Internet, or interface with the Internet, to transmit HCFA Privacy Act-protected and/or other sensitive HCFA information, including Virtual Private Network (VPN) and tunneling implementations over the Internet. Non-Internet Medicare/Medicaid data communications processes (e.g., use of private or value added networks) are not changed or affected by the Internet Policy. This policy covers Internet data transmission only. *It does not cover local data-at-rest or local host or network protections. Sensitive data-at-rest must still be protected by all necessary measures, in conformity with the guidelines/rules which govern the entity's possession of the data. Entities must use due diligence in exercising this responsibility.* Local site networks must also be protected against attack and penetration from the Internet with the use of firewalls and other protections. Such protective measures are outside the scope of this document, but are essential to providing adequate local security for data and the local networks and ADP systems which support it.

7. Acceptable Methods

HCFA Privacy Act–protected and/or other sensitive HCFA information sent over the Internet must be accessed only by authorized parties. Technologies that allow users to prove they are who they say they are (authentication or identification) and the organized scrambling of data (encryption) to avoid inappropriate disclosure or modification must be used to insure that data travels safely over the Internet and is only disclosed to authorized parties. Encryption must be at a sufficient level of security to protect against the cipher being readily broken and the data compromised. The length of the key and the quality of the encryption framework and algorithm must be increased over time as new weaknesses are discovered and processing power increases.

User authentication or identification must be coupled with the encryption and data transmission processes to be certain that confidential data is delivered only to authorized parties. There are a number of effective means for authentication or identification which are sufficiently trustworthy to be used, including both in-band authentication and out-of-band identification methods. Passwords may be sent over the Internet only when encrypted.[1]

Encryption Models and Approaches

Figure 1 depicts three generalized configurations of connectivity to the Internet. The generic model is not intended to be a literal mirror of the actual Internet interface configuration, but is intended to show that the encryption process takes place prior to information being presented to the Internet for transmission, and the decryption process after reception from the Internet. A large organization would be very likely to have the Internet Server/Gateway on their premises, while a small organization would likely have only the Internet Client, eg, a browser, on premises with the Internet Server at an Internet Service Provider (ISP). The Small User and Large User examples offer a more detailed depiction of the functional relationships involved.

The Encryption/Decryption process depicted graphically represents a number of different approaches. This process could involve encryption of files prior to transmittal, or it could be implemented through hardware or software functionality. The diagram does not intend to dictate how the process is to be accomplished, only that it must take place prior to introduction to the Internet. The "Boundary" on the diagrams represents the point at which security control passes from the local user. It lies on the user side of the Internet Server and may be at a local site or at an Internet Service Provider depending upon the configuration.

---

[1] *We note that the Health Insurance Portability and Accountability Act of 1966 (HIPAA) calls for stringent security protection for electronic health information both while maintained and while in transmission. The proposed Security Standard called for by HIPAA was published in the* Federal Register *on August 12, 1998. The public had until October 13, 1998, to comment on the proposed regulation. Based on public comments, a final regulation is planned for late 1999. Policy guidance contained in this bulletin is consistent with the proposed HIPAA security requirements.*

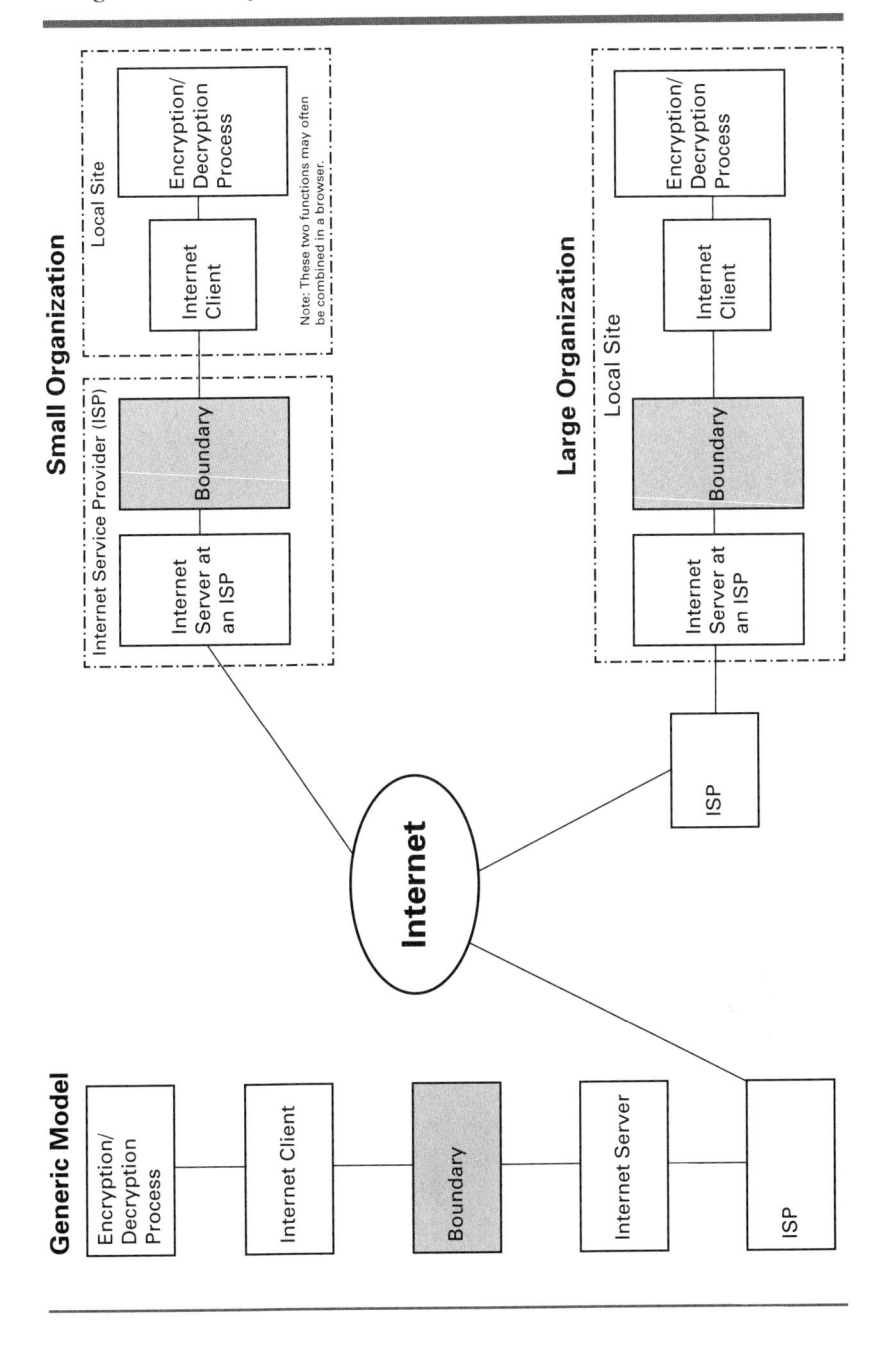

Using the Internet for Health Information: Legal Issues 59

Acceptable Approaches to Internet Usage

The method(s) employed by all users of HCFA Privacy Act-protected and/or other sensitive HCFA information must come under one of the approaches to encryption and at least one of the authentication or identification approaches. The use of multiple authentication or identification approaches is also permissible. These approaches are as generic as possible and as open to specific implementations as possible, to provide maximum user flexibility within the allowable limits of security and manageability.

Note the distinction that is made between the processes of "authentication" and "identification." In this Internet Policy, the terms "Authentication" and "Identification" are used in the following sense. They should not be interpreted as terms of art from any other source. Authentication refers to generally automated and formalized methods of establishing the authorized nature of a communications partner over the Internet communications data channel itself, generally called an "in-band process." Identification refers to less formal methods of establishing the authorized nature of a communications partner, which are usually manual, involve human interaction, and do not use the Internet data channel itself, but another "out-of-band" path such as the telephone or US mail.

The listed approaches provide encryption and authentication/identification techniques which are acceptable for use in safeguarding HCFA Privacy Act-protected and/or other sensitive HCFA information when it is transmitted over the Internet.

In summary, a complete Internet communications implementation must include *adequate encryption*, employment of *authentication or identification* of communications partners, and a management scheme to incorporate *effective password/key management* systems.

Acceptable Encryption Approaches

Note: As of November 1998, a level of encryption protection equivalent to that provided by an algorithm such as Triple 56 bit DES (defined as 112 bit equivalent) for symmetric encryption, 1024 bit algorithms for asymmetric systems, and 160 bits for the emerging Elliptical Curve systems is recognized by HCFA as minimally acceptable. HCFA reserves the right to increase these minimum levels when deemed necessary by advances in techniques and capabilities associated with the processes used by attackers to break encryption (for example, a brute-force exhaustive search).

Hardware-based Encryption

1. Hardware encryptors—While likely to be reserved for the largest traffic volumes to a very limited number of Internet sites, such symmetric password "private" key devices (such as link encryptors) are acceptable.

Software-based Encryption

2. Secure Sockets Layer (SSL) (Sometimes referred to as Transport Layer Security—TLS) implementations—At a minimum SSL level of Version 3.0, standard commercial implementations of PKI, or some variation thereof, implemented in the Secure Sockets Layer are acceptable.
3. S-MIME—Standard commercial implementations of encryption in the e-mail layer are acceptable.
4. In-stream—Encryption implementations in the transport layer, such as pre-agreed passwords, are acceptable.
5. Offline—Encryption/decryption of files at the user sites before entering the data communications process is acceptable. These encrypted files would then be attached

to or enveloped (tunneled) within an unencrypted header and/or transmission.

Acceptable Authentication Approaches

AUTHENTICATION (This function is accomplished over the Internet, and is referred to as an "in-band" process.)

1. Formal Certificate Authority-based use of digital certificates is acceptable.
2. Locally managed digital certificates are acceptable, providing all parties to the communication are covered by the certificates.
3. Self-authentication, as in internal control of symmetric "private" keys, is acceptable.
4. Tokens or "smart cards" are acceptable for authentication. In-band tokens involve overall network control of the token database for all parties.

Acceptable Identification Approaches

IDENTIFICATION (The process of identification takes place outside of the Internet connection and is referred to as an "out-of-band" process.)

1. Telephonic identification of users and/or password exchange is acceptable. Exchange of passwords and identities by US Certified Mail is acceptable.
2. Exchange of passwords and identities by bonded messenger is acceptable.
3. Direct personal contact exchange of passwords and identities between users is acceptable.
4. Tokens or "smart cards" are acceptable for identification. Out-of-band tokens involve local control of the token databases with the local authenticated server vouching for specific local users.

8. Requirements and Audits

Each organization that uses the Internet to transmit HCFA Privacy Act-protected and/or other sensitive HCFA information will be expected to meet the stated requirements set forth in this document. All organizations subject to OMB Circular A-130 are required to have a Security Plan. All such organizations must modify their Security Plan to detail the methodologies and protective measures if they decide to use the Internet for transmittal of HCFA Privacy Act-protected and/or other sensitive HCFA information, and to adequately test implemented measures. HCFA reserves the right to audit any organization's implementation of, and/or adherence to the requirements, as stated in this policy. This includes the right to require that any organization utilizing the Internet for transmission of HCFA Privacy Act-protected and/or other sensitive information submit documentation to demonstrate that they meet these requirements.

9. Acknowledgement of Intent

Organizations desiring to use the Internet for transmittal of HCFA Privacy Act-protected and/or other sensitive HCFA information must notify HCFA of this intent. An e-mail address is provided below to be used for this acknowledgment. An acknowledgment must include the following information:

> Name of Organization
> Address of Organization
> Type/Nature of Information being transmitted
> Name of Contact (eg, CIO or accountable official)
> Contact's telephone number and e-mail address

For submission of acknowledgment of intent, send an e-mail to: internetsecurity@hcfa.gov. Internal HCFA elements must proceed through the usual HCFA system and project development process.

10. Point of Contact

For questions or comment, write to:
    Office of Information Services, HCFA
    Security and Standards Group
    Division of HCFA Enterprise Standards-Internet
    7500 Security Boulevard
    Baltimore, MD 21244

Appendix C

Disclaimer Used on America's Doctor Web Site

This form disclaimer is provided for informational purposes only and is not intended as legal advice. Copies of this disclaimer may only be made with the prior permission of America's Doctor, Inc.

Welcome to America's Doctor Chat!

Before you meet your America's Doctor, you need to complete two important steps. First, read the terms of service, below. You need to understand our terms, and agree to them, before chatting with your America's Doctor. Next, let us know how we can help you today. By selecting a topic from the list on the next page, you'll be assured of seeing the best America's Doctor for your needs.

1. Disclaimer on Emergency Medical Conditions

DO NOT USE THIS SITE FOR MEDICAL EMERGENCY SERVICES. IN AN EMERGENCY, CALL 911 OR YOUR LOCAL EMERGENCY ASSISTANCE NUMBER.

Source: America's Doctor Inc. Welcome to America's Doctor chat. America's Doctor™ Online Web site. Available at:
http://www.americasdoctor.com/askadoc/master_frame.htm.
Accessed April 13, 1999. Used with permission.

2. General Disclaimers About Our Physicians and Sponsor Hospitals

America's Doctor is one way for you to gather general medical information and to make contact with certain hospitals in your area who have arranged to make information available through our Web site. By clicking on the button below, marked "accept," you acknowledge that you have reviewed and agree to all of the above provisions, disclosures and disclaimers. America's Doctor Inc. reserves the right to modify or supplement any or all of them, and they shall continue to apply, as modified, to each user's current, prior or subsequent use of this Web site. The application of these provisions, disclosures and disclaimers and all other matters arising from your use of this Web site or of any information you obtain from America's Doctor shall be governed by the laws of the United States of America and the State of Maryland. Any claims, disputes or other controversies relating to or arising from these provisions, disclosures and disclaimers or from your use of this Web site or any information you receive from America's Doctor shall be brought exclusively in the United States District Court, Maryland District, Baltimore Division or the Circuit Court for Baltimore County, Maryland, and you hereby expressly consent to the exercise of jurisdiction over you by such courts. To the fullest extent permitted by applicable law, each party to this Agreement waives its or his right to a jury trial with respect to any action brought under or in connection with this Agreement. Any notice to America's Doctor shall be given in writing and sent by certified and registered mail to America's Doctor Inc., 11403 Cronridge Drive, Suite 200, Owings Mills MD 21117, Attn: CEO, President.

---

* You must be at least 18 years of age to use America's Doctor and agree not to post any information which (a) is libelous, defamatory, obscene, fraudulent, false or contrary to the ownership or intellectual property rights of any other person, or (b) contains any virus, worm, Trojan horse or other code which is contaminating or destructive to the files or programs of America's Doctor or any of its users.

Our Staff

Our staff includes physicians. None of our physicians will enter into a physician-patient relationship with you. They can assist you in your personal, general research but they will not engage in any conduct that involves the practice of medicine. The information you obtain from America's Doctor should not substitute or be used instead of a relationship with a health care professional. All users are encouraged to seek the advice of, and regularly consult with, physicians and other health care professionals of their selection.

In addition to physicians, our staff includes other medical practitioners including, without limitation, pharmacists, nutritionists, nurses, nurse practitioners, and other health care professionals. None of these other health care professionals are engaged to provide health care services to you and should not be considered to be in a clinical or treatment relationship with you. Rather, like our physicians, these professionals are available solely to assist you in your research. Professionals engaged by America's Doctor will not retain any records, monitor your care or establish a confidential patient relationship with you. None of these other practitioners on our staff should be considered to be your treating or caregiving health care professional and will not communicate with your own health care provider. Consequently, the information you obtain from America's Doctor should not substitute or be used instead of a relationship with a health care professional. All users are encouraged to seek the advice of, and regularly consult with, physicians and other health care professionals of their selection.

America's Doctor establishes requirements for the credentials of our physicians, including the requirement that they be "Board-certified" or "Board-eligible" in a particular specialty, but we reserve the discretion whether to change or waive these requirements. Our physicians are not practicing medicine or providing medical advice or opinions to you. Thus, these credentials are solely for our benefit.

Our physicians do not (a) diagnose, (b) treat, or (c) prescribe for anyone using our Web site.

Our physicians will not accept payment from you and will not bill any insurance company, government payment program or other source of health benefits.

If you contact our Web site more than once, you are not guaranteed that you will be put in contact with the same physician and you may not request to be put in contact with the same physician.

Our physicians are instructed not to contact any caller outside of the immediate, on-line question and answer session. Even if you give your name and any contact information to one of our physicians, none of our physicians will contact you for follow-up. They will not communicate with your personal physician or any other health care provider.

Our physicians do not keep any medical records and will not have any records concerning prior contacts you may have made to our Web site.

Please do not share personal medical information of a kind you would wish to be held confidential. Since our physicians are not in a physician-patient relationship with you, the information you provide will not be considered a medical record. While America's Doctor does not sell medical information, we may provide general aggregate information about our users to our Sponsor Hospitals. While America's Doctor attempts, along with AOL, to prevent unauthorized persons from accessing our files or tampering with our site, we cannot guarantee that these efforts will always be successful. America's Doctor shall have the right to use any questions, comments, or other information submitted by users in books, articles, commentaries, research or similar ways.

If you decide to seek information or obtain treatment from any of our sponsor hospitals, our physicians will not follow up or monitor your care.

Our Sponsor Hospitals

America's Doctor has agreements with various hospitals, which we call our "Sponsor Hospitals." Sponsor Hospitals have made arrangements with us to post advertisements on our Web site. These advertisements may appear based on the zip code where you reside.

Our relationships with a Sponsor Hospital in a particular area are based on factors we establish, which may include offering exclusivity in a particular region based on a first-come, first-contracted response.

We contract with our Sponsor Hospitals for a monthly fee. This fee is not based on the volume or value of any services Sponsor Hospitals may or may not provide to our users.

We do not endorse or credential the services our Sponsor Hospitals advertise and make no representations or warranties about the type of services, quality of care, source of payment or billing practices of our Sponsor Hospitals. We are not a service that verifies and updates the licenses, accreditations, certifications or other permits and approvals of any Sponsor Hospital.

If you indicate that you wish information about or from a Sponsor Hospital, or to be contacted by a Sponsor Hospital, this information is passed along to the Sponsor Hospital. We also provide general information about the users who contact our Web site to our Sponsor Hospitals.

If you desire information about a hospital in your area which is not a Sponsor Hospital, we will try to provide you with that information. If we are unable to provide you with the specific information requested, we may instead provide you with a more general, local resource that can direct you further about other hospitals.

Information From Others

America's Doctor may include or provide links to other Web sites on the Internet, including, but not limited to, links to sponsor hospitals' Web pages and online volunteer studies, which may include information, opinions or recommendations of various individuals, organizations or companies. America's Doctor has no affiliation with such Web sites or the individuals, organizations or companies responsible for them. In providing such links, America's Doctor does not represent to you that it has investigated the content of such information, opinions or recommendations and thus you understand and agree that America's Doctor does not warrant or guarantee the accuracy of such information or necessarily subscribe to any such opinions or recommendations. Further, to the extent that you make use of any link to any other Web site on the Internet which is made available to you, you hereby agree that you will not reproduce, sell or distribute information contained in the study or disclose such information to others.

Our Information

America's Doctor strives to be a valuable resource of timely information for our users. We cannot ensure that information we provide is exhaustive or complete on every subject or that it will necessarily include all of the most recent information available on a particular topic. This information is of a general nature and we urge you to review it with your attending physician. Users should never delay, ignore or fail to obtain medical advice based on information obtained from America's Doctor.

3. Copyright and Trademark

All text and images Copyright ©1998 by America's Doctor, Inc. The name "America's Doctor" and associated logo are proprietary trademarks and service marks of America's Doctor, Inc.

America's Doctor, Inc.'s materials may be downloaded by users for personal use only. Permission to otherwise reprint or electronically reproduce any America's Doctor materials is expressly prohibited without prior written consent from America's Doctor, Inc. Users shall not provide copyrighted or other proprietary information to America's Doctor without permission from the owner of such material or rights and shall be solely responsible for any damages resulting from such disclosures. Users shall be solely responsible for obtaining such permission.

4. Miscellaneous

When we receive an e-mail, we make reasonable efforts to respond in as timely a manner as possible but we cannot represent or warrant how quickly we will be able to respond and you should not refrain from seeking medical treatment while waiting for information from us.

INFORMATION SUPPLIED BY AMERICA'S DOCTOR IS PROVIDED "AS IS" AND NEITHER AMERICA'S DOCTOR NOR ANY OF OUR STAFF, INCLUDING WITHOUT LIMITATION OUR PHYSICIANS AND SPONSOR HOSPITALS, MAKE ANY REPRESENTATION OR WARRANTY WITH RESPECT TO THE CONTENTS OF THIS WEB SITE OR INFORMATION FURNISHED BY THEM OR OUR AGENTS, EMPLOYEES OR REPRESENTATIVES AND SPECIFICALLY DISCLAIM TO THE FULLEST EXTENT PERMITTED BY LAW ANY AND ALL WARRANTIES, EXPRESS OR IMPLIED, INCLUDING, BUT NOT LIMITED TO, IMPLIED WARRANTIES OF MERCHANTABILITY, COMPLETENESS, TIMELINESS, CORRECTNESS, NONINFRINGEMENT, OR FITNESS FOR ANY PARTICULAR USE, APPLICATION OR PURPOSE. YOU HEREBY ALSO AGREE THAT AMERICA'S DOCTOR, AND ITS OFFICERS, DIRECTORS, AGENTS AND EMPLOYEES, SHALL NOT BE LIABLE TO YOU FOR ANY DAMAGES, CLAIMS, DEMANDS OR CAUSES OF ACTION, DIRECT OR INDIRECT, SPECIAL, INCIDENTAL, CONSEQUENTIAL OR PUNITIVE, AS A RESULT OF YOUR USE OF THIS WEB SITE OR ANY INFORMATION YOU OBTAIN ON IT OR ANY OTHER INTERACTION WITH AMERICA'S DOCTOR. IN DOING SO, YOU AGREE THAT YOU ARE WAIVING VOLUNTARILY AND UNEQUIVOCALLY ANY LIABILITY OF AMERICA'S DOCTOR.

America's Doctor cannot make any representation or warranty concerning errors, omissions, delays or other defects in the information supplied to users, or that its files are free of viruses, worms, Trojan horses or other code that include or manifest contaminating or destructive characteristics.

America's Doctor does not guarantee that it will respond to all inquiries and reserves the right to ignore or delete any information including, without limitation, information that is fraudulent, abusive, defamatory, obscene or in violation of a copyright, trademark or other intellectual property or ownership right of any other person.

If any clause or provision set forth above is determined to be illegal, invalid or unenforceable under present or future law, then, in that event, you understand and agree that the clause or provision so determined to be illegal, invalid or unenforceable shall be severable without affecting the enforceability of all remaining clauses or provisions.

You acknowledge that the provisions, disclosures and disclaimers set forth above are fair and reasonable and your agreement to follow and be bound to them is not the result of fraud, duress or undue influence exercised upon you by any person or entity. There are no representations, promises, warranties or undertakings by America's Doctor contrary to those set forth above. By clicking on the button below marked "accept" you acknowledge that you have reviewed and agree to all of the above provisions, disclosures and disclaimers. Any notice to America's Doctor shall be given in writing and sent by certified and registered mail to America's Doctor Inc., 11403 Cronridge Drive, Suite 200, Owings Mills MD 21117, Attn: CEO.

Appendix D

Disclaimer Used by Mayo Clinic

This form disclaimer is provided for informational purposes only and is not intended as legal advice.

Online Service Agreement

Mayo Clinic Health Oasis (the "Service") is an online information and communications service provided by Mayo Foundation for Medical Education and Research ("Provider") subject to your agreement with all of the terms and conditions offered below. Please read this Agreement carefully before accessing or using the Service. By accessing or using the Service, you agree to be bound by all of the terms and conditions below, which are intended to be fully effective and binding upon the Provider and users. The Provider may modify this Agreement at any time, and such modifications shall be effective immediately upon posting the modified Agreement. You agree to review the Agreement periodically to be aware of such modifications and your accessing or using the Service constitutes your acceptance of the Agreement as it appears at the time of your access or use.

THE INFORMATION CONTAINED IN THIS SERVICE IS NOT INTENDED NOR IMPLIED TO BE A SUBSTITUTE FOR PROFESSIONAL MEDICAL ADVICE. ALWAYS SEEK THE ADVICE OF YOUR PHYSICIAN OR OTHER QUALIFIED HEALTH PROVIDER PRIOR TO STARTING ANY NEW TREATMENT OR WITH ANY QUESTIONS

Source: Mayo Foundation for Medical Education and Research. Online service agreement. Mayo Clinic Health Oasis Web site. Available at: http://www.mayohealth.org/mayo/common/htm/disclaim.htm. Accessed April 13, 1999. Used with permission.

YOU MAY HAVE REGARDING A MEDICAL CONDITION. NOTHING CONTAINED IN THE SERVICE IS INTENDED TO BE FOR MEDICAL DIAGNOSIS OR TREATMENT.

You understand that, except for information, products or services clearly identified as being supplied by the Provider, the Provider does not operate, control or endorse any information, products or services on the Internet, including on the Service, in any way. You also understand that the Provider cannot and does not guarantee or warrant that files available for downloading through the Service will be free of infection or viruses, worms, Trojan horses or other code that manifest contaminating or destructive properties. Each Member is responsible for implementing sufficient procedures and checkpoints to satisfy his or her particular requirements for accuracy of data input and output, and for maintaining a means external to the Service for the reconstruction of any lost data. The Provider does not assume any responsibility or risk for your use of the Service.

THE PROVIDER DOES NOT MAKE ANY EXPRESS OR IMPLIED WARRANTIES, REPRESENTATIONS OR ENDORSEMENTS WHATSOEVER (INCLUDING WITHOUT LIMITATION WARRANTIES OF TITLE OR NONINFRINGEMENT, OR THE IMPLIED WARRANTIES OF MERCHANTABILITY OR FITNESS FOR A PARTICULAR PURPOSE) WITH REGARD TO THE SERVICE, ANY MERCHANDISE, INFORMATION OR SERVICE PROVIDED THROUGH THE SERVICE. EXCEPT AS OTHERWISE EXPRESSLY SPECIFIED, THE PROVIDER DOES NOT WARRANT THE ACCURACY, COMPLETENESS OR CORRECTNESS, TIMELINESS, OR USEFULNESS OF ANY OPINIONS, ADVICE, SERVICES, MERCHANDISE OR OTHER INFORMATION PROVIDED THROUGH THE SERVICE OR ON THE INTERNET GENERALLY. IN NO EVENT WILL THE PROVIDER BE LIABLE TO YOU OR ANYONE ELSE FOR ANY DECISION MADE OR ACTION TAKEN BY YOU OR ANYONE ELSE IN RELIANCE UPON THE INFORMATION PROVIDED THROUGH THE SERVICE.

With regard to USP information on this site:

- The information about drugs contained in this database is general in nature and is intended for use as an educational aid. It does not cover all possible uses, actions, precautions, side effects, or interactions of these medicines, nor is the information intended as medical advice for individual problems or for making an evaluation as to the risks and benefits of taking a particular drug.

- The information in these leaflets has been selectively abstracted from USP DI® for use as an educational aid and does not cover all possible uses, actions, precautions, side effects, or interactions of this medicine. It is not intended as medical advice for individual problems.

- The text that a user may be viewing at any one time, or may print, may contain only a portion of the full Leaflet or USP monograph. The entire USP DI® should be consulted for complete information.

- NOTICE: The information provided by the USP Convention contained herein has been devised without reference to cultural, dietary, societal, language, prescribing or dispensing conditions (including those imposed by law), other than those of the United States, which might affect the information provided.

- Information is for personal use only and may not be sold or redistributed.

The Service is presented by the Provider for the sole purpose of disseminating health information for public benefit. IT IS NOT INTENDED, AND MUST NOT BE TAKEN, TO BE THE PROVISION OR PRACTICE OF MEDICAL, NURSING, OR PROFESSIONAL HEALTH CARE ADVICE OR SERVICES IN ANY JURISDICTION.

THE SERVICE IS NOT TARGETED TO USERS IN ANY PARTICULAR LOCALITY, NOR IS IT INTENDED TO CONSTITUTE THE DOING OF BUSINESS IN ANY JURISDICTION, NOR TO BE A SOLICITATION OF BUSINESS ANYWHERE ON BEHALF OF MAYO CLINIC OR ANY OF ITS AFFILIATED CORPORATIONS, NOR TO CONSTITUTE ANY CONTACTS WITH ANY JURISDICTION OUTSIDE OF THE STATE OF MINNESOTA.

Potential users in any jurisdiction in the world, the common, statutory, regulatory, or codified law of which would void this Agreement in whole or in any essential part (the essential parts being at least, but not only, the exclusive venue and exclusive remedy provisions, and warranty disclaimer), or which makes accessing the Service illegal, are unauthorized to use the Service, and do so entirely at their own risk.

IN NO EVENT SHALL THE PROVIDER BE LIABLE FOR ANY DIRECT, INDIRECT, INCIDENTAL, CONSEQUENTIAL, SPECIAL, EXEMPLARY, PUNITIVE, OR ANY OTHER MONETARY OR OTHER DAMAGES, FEES, FINES, PENALTIES, OR LIABILITIES ARISING OUT OF OR RELATING IN ANY WAY TO THIS SERVICE, OR SITES ACCESSED THROUGH THIS SERVICE, AND/OR CONTENT OR INFORMATION PROVIDED HEREIN. A USER'S SOLE AND EXCLUSIVE REMEDY FOR DISSATISFACTION WITH THE SERVICE IS TO STOP USING THE SERVICE.

This Agreement is entered into and performed in the State of Minnesota, United States of America, and is governed by and shall be construed in all respects under the laws of Minnesota, exclusive of its choice of law or conflict of laws provisions. In any claim or action directly or indirectly arising under this Agreement or related to the Service, each party irrevocably submits to the exclusive personal jurisdiction of the Minnesota State District Court sitting in Olmsted County, Minnesota, or if such court does not have subject-matter jurisdiction, then each party irrevocably submits to the exclusive personal jurisdiction of the United States Court for the District of Minnesota, and whichever of those two courts has jurisdiction, each party waives any jurisdictional, venue, or inconvenient forum objections to such court.

If any of the provisions of this Agreement are held by a court or other tribunal of competent jurisdiction not to be enforceable, then such provisions shall be limited or eliminated to the minimum extent necessary so that this Agreement shall otherwise remain in full force and effect. This Agreement constitutes the entire agreement between the parties pertaining to its subject matter. It may not be modified except as described elsewhere in this Agreement. Anything in the Service inconsistent with or conflicting with the terms of this Agreement is superseded by the terms of this Agreement.

The marks "Mayo Clinic Health Oasis," "Mayo," "Mayo Clinic," the triple-shield Mayo logo and "Reliable Information for a Healthier Life" are used under license by Mayo Foundation for Medical Education and Research. "USP DI and Advice for the Patient" are registered trademarks of the United States Pharmacopeial Convention, Inc.

The materials on Our Service are copyrighted by the respective Provider and may be downloaded and/or reprinted for personal use only. Permission to reprint or electronically reproduce any document or graphic in whole or in part for any reason is expressly prohibited, unless prior written consent is obtained from the respective copyright holder(s).

> I accept all of the foregoing terms either by clicking here or by any further use of the Service.

> I do not accept all of the foregoing terms.